The Healthy Gout Diet Cookbook

Delectable Dishes to Overcome Gout and Enjoy a Life Free from Pain

EMMANUEL AKINNODI

TABLE OF CONTENTS

14. Baked Cauliflower Rice Casserole

15. Lemon Herb Roasted Chicken Thighs

16. Mediterranean Chickpea Salad

17. Zucchini Noodles with Pesto Sauce

18. Stuffed Mushrooms with Spinach and Goat Cheese

19. Citrus and Herb Baked Tilapia

20. Lentil and Quinoa Stuffed Bell Peppers

21. Chicken and Vegetable Curry

22. Roasted Asparagus with Lemon and Parmesan

23. Shrimp and Avocado Salad

24. Cauliflower Crust Margherita Pizza

25. Berry and Spinach Smoothie

CONCLUSION

INTRODUCTION

My name is John, and I was diagnosed with gout a few years ago. I had been experiencing severe pain in my big toe, and the doctor told me that it was caused by high levels of uric acid in my blood. He put me on medication, but the pain didn't go away. I was starting to feel really depressed and hopeless.

One day, I was browsing the bookstore and I saw a book called "The Gout Diet Cookbook." I picked it up and started reading, and I was amazed by how much information it contained. The book explained what gout is, how it's caused, and how to prevent it. It also included a whole chapter of delicious recipes that were low in purines, which are the substances that can trigger gout attacks.

I decided to give the diet a try, and I was really surprised by how well it worked. Within a few weeks, the pain in my toe had started to subside. I kept following the diet, and eventually the pain went away completely. I was so happy!

I've been following the diet for a few years now, and I haven't had a gout attack since. I feel so much better now, and I'm so grateful to the author of the Gout Diet Cookbook for helping me turn my life around.

I'm so glad that I found the book, and I hope that my story will help other people who are struggling with gout. If you're reading this and you're feeling hopeless, please don't give up. There is hope, and there is a way to manage your gout and live a normal life.

Gout is a painful condition that affects millions of people around the world. It is caused by high levels of uric acid in the blood, which can form crystals in the joints. These crystals can cause inflammation and pain, which can be severe.

The Healthy Gout Diet Cookbook is a comprehensive guide to help you manage your gout and live a healthier life. This cookbook offers a wide array of delicious and flavorful dishes that are low in purines, the substances that can trigger gout attacks.

Each recipe is carefully crafted to be both delicious and nutritious, so you can enjoy the foods you love without sacrificing your health. This cookbook offers a wide array of delectable dishes that not only soothe gout symptoms but also ignite a passion for flavorful, healthy eating.

From appetizers bursting with flavor to main courses that tantalize the palate and divine desserts that bring a sweet finale to every meal, each dish is infused with love and thoughtfulness to nourish your body and soul. Embracing a healthier lifestyle has never been more enjoyable and empowering.

With this book as your guide, you'll not only conquer gout but also embark on a journey of transformation, breaking free from the confines of pain and embracing a life of joy, vitality, and flavorful living. With The Healthy Gout Diet Cookbook, you have everything you need to take control of your gout and live a pain-free life. So what are you waiting for? Start cooking today!

So, join us on this extraordinary culinary adventure, where every page is a step toward reclaiming your wellbeing and relishing every moment free from pain. With" The Healthy Gout Diet Cookbook", you have everything you need to take control of your gout and live a pain-free life. So what are you waiting for? Start cooking today!

25 EASY, QUICK AND DELICIOUS GOUT DIET RECIPES

1. Quinoa and Roasted Vegetable Salad:

Ingredients:

1 cup quinoa, rinsed

A variety of vegetables (bell peppers, zucchini, and cherry tomatoes)

2 tablespoons olive oil

2 tablespoons balsamic vinegar

Fresh basil leaves

Salt and pepper to taste

Preparation:

Cook quinoa according to package instructions.

Toss vegetables with olive oil, salt, and pepper. Roast in the oven at 400°F (200°C) until tender.

Combine cooked quinoa and roasted vegetables. Drizzle them with the delightful tang of balsamic vinegar, topping it all off with a sprinkling of fresh basil leaves.

2. Lemon Herb Grilled Chicken:

Ingredients:

4 boneless, skinless chicken breasts

2 tablespoons olive oil

Juice and zest of 1 lemon

2 cloves garlic, minced

1 tablespoon fresh thyme leaves

Salt and pepper to taste

Preparation:

In a bowl, mix olive oil, lemon juice, zest, minced garlic, thyme, salt, and pepper.

Marinate chicken breasts in the mixture for at least 30 minutes.

Achieve grilled perfection with the chicken, cooking it over a gentle flame until it reaches its deliciously tender, fully cooked state.

3. Baked Salmon with Dill Sauce:

Ingredients:

4 salmon fillets

2 tablespoons olive oil

2 tablespoons fresh dill, chopped

Juice of 1 lemon

Salt and pepper to taste

Preparation:

Preheat oven to 375°F (190°C).

Place salmon fillets on a baking sheet. Drizzle with olive oil, lemon juice, and sprinkle with dill, salt, and pepper.

Let the oven work its magic as you bake the salmon for 15-20 minutes, ensuring it emerges perfectly cooked and ready to savor.

4. Lentil and Vegetable Soup:

Ingredients:

1 cup dried lentils

1 onion, diced

2 carrots, diced

2 celery stalks, diced

2 cloves garlic, minced

4 cups vegetable broth

1 bay leaf

1 teaspoon dried thyme

Salt and pepper to taste

Preparation:

Rinse lentils and set aside.

Begin your culinary journey by sautéing a trio of onions, carrots, and celery in a large pot until they reach a softened, fragrant state. Stir in garlic to add an extra layer of flavor.

Add lentils, vegetable broth, bay leaf, thyme, salt, and pepper.

Allow the flavors to mingle and meld as you bring the mixture to a gentle boil, then gracefully lower the heat and let it simmer for a blissful 30-40 minutes.

5. Grilled Portobello Mushrooms with Balsamic Glaze:

Ingredients:

4 large portobello mushrooms

3 tablespoons balsamic vinegar

1 tablespoon olive oil

2 cloves garlic, minced

Fresh parsley for garnish

Salt and pepper to taste

Preparation:

Preheat grill to medium-high heat.

In a bowl, mix balsamic vinegar, olive oil, minced garlic, salt, and pepper.

Brush mushroom caps with the mixture and grill for 5-7 minutes per side.

Garnish with fresh parsley before serving.

6. Spinach and Strawberry Salad with Poppy Seed Dressing:

Ingredients:

4 cups baby spinach

1 cup strawberries, sliced

1/4 cup sliced almonds

2 tablespoons poppy seeds

1 tablespoon honey

2 tablespoons apple cider vinegar

2 tablespoons olive oil

Preparation:

Craft a refreshing and delightful salad by combining tender baby spinach with the sweet allure of sliced strawberries.

In a separate bowl, whisk together poppy seeds, honey, apple cider vinegar, and olive oil to make the dressing.

Drizzle dressing over the salad and sprinkle with sliced almonds.

7. Turkey and Vegetable Stir-Fry:

Ingredients:

1 pound turkey breast, thinly sliced

2 cups broccoli florets

1 red bell pepper, sliced

1 tablespoon sesame oil

2 tablespoons low-sodium soy sauce

2 cloves garlic, minced

1 tablespoon grated ginger

1 tablespoon cornstarch

1/4 cup water

Sesame seeds for garnish

Preparation:

Embark on an Asian-inspired culinary adventure by heating sesame oil to sizzling perfection in a wok or large skillet over medium-high heat.

Add turkey slices, garlic, and ginger. Cook until the turkey is browned.

Add broccoli and bell pepper, and stir-fry for a few minutes until tender-crisp.

In a small bowl, mix soy sauce, cornstarch, and water. Pour over the stir-fry and cook until the sauce thickens.

Garnish with sesame seeds before serving.

8. *Stuffed Bell Peppers with Quinoa and Black Beans:*

Ingredients:

4 large bell peppers, seeded and cut in half.

1 cup cooked quinoa

1 can (15 oz) washed and drained black beans

1 cup diced tomatoes

1 teaspoon chili powder

1 teaspoon cumin

1/2 cup shredded cheddar cheese (optional)

Fresh cilantro for garnish

Salt and pepper to taste

Preparation:

Preheat the oven to 375°F (190°C).

In a bowl, mix cooked quinoa, black beans, diced tomatoes, chili powder, cumin, salt, and pepper.

Stuff each half of the bell pepper with the delightful quinoa mixture.

Place stuffed bell peppers on a baking sheet and bake for 20-25 minutes.

If desired, top with shredded cheddar cheese and bake for an additional 5 minutes until melted.

Garnish with fresh cilantro before serving.

9. Baked Sweet Potatoes with Avocado Salsa:

Ingredients:

4 medium sweet potatoes

2 avocados, diced

1/4 cup diced red onion

1 jalapeño, seeded and minced

Juice of 1 lime

Fresh cilantro for garnish

Salt and pepper to taste

Preparation:

Preheat the oven to 400°F (200°C).

Allow the sweet potatoes to bake for 45-60 minutes or until they become tender.

In a bowl, mix diced avocados, red onion, jalapeño, lime juice, salt, and pepper to make the salsa.

Cut open baked sweet potatoes and top with avocado salsa. Garnish with fresh cilantro.

10. Lemon Garlic Shrimp Skewers:

Ingredients:

1 pound of peeled and deveined big shrimp

2 tablespoons olive oil

Zest and juice of 1 lemon

3 cloves garlic, minced

1 teaspoon dried oregano

Salt and pepper to taste

Preparation:

In a bowl, mix olive oil, lemon zest, lemon juice, minced garlic, oregano, salt, and pepper.

Marinate shrimp in the mixture for 15-30 minutes.

Skewer the shrimp and grill them over medium-high heat for approximately 2-3 minutes per side until they are thoroughly cooked.

11. Quinoa Stuffed Acorn Squash:

Ingredients:

2 acorn squash, cut in half, with seeds removed

1 cup cooked quinoa

1 cup chopped kale

1/2 cup dried cranberries

1/4 cup chopped pecans

1 tablespoon maple syrup

Preparation:

Preheat the oven to 400°F (200°C).

Place acorn squash halves on a baking sheet, cut side down, and roast for 20 minutes.

In a bowl, mix cooked quinoa, chopped kale, dried cranberries, chopped pecans, and maple syrup.

Remove the squash from the oven and flip them over. Stuff the quinoa mixture into each hollow squash half.

Return to the oven and bake for an additional 15-20 minutes until the squash is tender.

12. Grilled Eggplant and Tomato Stack:

Ingredients:

1 large eggplant, sliced into rounds

2 large tomatoes, sliced

1 cup fresh mozzarella slices

Fresh basil leaves

Balsamic glaze

Olive oil

Salt and pepper to taste

Preparation:

Coat the eggplant slices with olive oil, then sprinkle with salt and pepper.

Grill eggplant slices for 3-4 minutes per side until tender.

Layer grilled eggplant, tomato slices, and fresh mozzarella to create stacks.

Add a drizzle of balsamic glaze and a sprinkle of fresh basil leaves as a finishing touch.

13. Cucumber and Avocado Gazpacho:

Ingredients:

2 large cucumbers, peeled and chopped

2 avocados, peeled and pitted

1/4 cup chopped red onion

2 cloves garlic, minced

2 tablespoons fresh lime juice

1 cup vegetable broth

Fresh dill for garnish

Salt and pepper to taste

Preparation:

In a blender, combine chopped cucumbers, avocados, red onion, minced garlic, lime juice, and vegetable broth.

Blend until smooth, adding more broth if needed for desired consistency.

Make sure to adjust the seasoning with salt and pepper according to your taste.

Give the dish some time to cool off in the fridge for a minimum of 30 minutes before you're ready to serve it.

Garnish with fresh dill before serving.

14. Baked Cauliflower Rice Casserole:

Ingredients:

4 cups cauliflower rice

1 cup of chopped, multicolored bell peppers

1 cup diced zucchini

1/2 cup diced red onion

1 cup shredded mozzarella cheese

1 cup low-sodium marinara sauce

2 tablespoons olive oil

1 tablespoon Italian seasoning

Salt and pepper to taste

Preparation:

Preheat the oven to 375°F (190°C).

In a large skillet, sauté diced bell peppers, zucchini, and red onion in olive oil until softened.

In a casserole dish, layer cauliflower rice, sautéed vegetables, marinara sauce, shredded mozzarella, Italian seasoning, salt, and pepper.

Layer the ingredients repeatedly until everything is used, and make sure the top is covered with a final layer of mozzarella.

Bake the dish until the cheese turns bubbly and golden, which typically takes 20-25 minutes.

15. Lemon Herb Roasted Chicken Thighs:

Ingredients:

4 chicken thighs, bone-in and skin-on

2 tablespoons olive oil

Juice and zest of 1 lemon

2 tablespoons chopped fresh rosemary

2 cloves garlic, minced

Salt and pepper to taste

Preparation:

Preheat the oven to 425°F (220°C).

In a bowl, mix olive oil, lemon juice, zest, chopped rosemary, minced garlic, salt, and pepper.

Place the chicken thighs in a baking dish and pour the marinade generously over them.

Roast in the oven for 30-35 minutes or until chicken is cooked through and skin is crispy.

16. Mediterranean Chickpea Salad:

Ingredients:

2 cups cooked chickpeas

1 cucumber, diced

1 pint cherry tomatoes, halved

1/2 cup chopped Kalamata olives

1/4 cup crumbled feta cheese (optional)

2 tablespoons fresh lemon juice

2 tablespoons olive oil

1 teaspoon dried oregano

Salt and pepper to taste

Preparation:

In a large bowl, combine cooked chickpeas, diced cucumber, halved cherry tomatoes, and chopped Kalamata olives.

If you prefer feta cheese, include it in the bowl of ingredients.

In a separate bowl, whisk together fresh lemon juice, olive oil, dried oregano, salt, and pepper to make the dressing.

Drizzle the dressing over the salad and give it a toss to coat everything evenly.

17. Zucchini Noodles with Pesto Sauce:

Ingredients:

4 medium zucchinis, spiralized into noodles

1 cup fresh basil leaves

1/4 cup grated Parmesan cheese

1/4 cup pine nuts

2 cloves garlic

1/4 cup olive oil

Juice of 1 lemon

Salt and pepper to taste

Preparation:

In a food processor, combine fresh basil leaves, grated Parmesan cheese, pine nuts, garlic, olive oil, lemon juice, salt, and pepper to make the pesto sauce.

In a large skillet, sauté the zucchini noodles until they reach a tender texture.

Toss zucchini noodles with pesto sauce and serve.

18. Stuffed Mushrooms with Spinach and Goat Cheese:

Ingredients:

12 big mushrooms, stems cut off and minced

2 cups chopped spinach

1/4 cup crumbled goat cheese

2 tablespoons olive oil

2 cloves garlic, minced

Salt and pepper to taste

Preparation:

Preheat the oven to 375°F (190°C).

In a skillet, sauté chopped mushroom stems and minced garlic in olive oil until softened.

Add chopped spinach to the skillet and cook until wilted.

Remove from heat and stir in crumbled goat cheese, salt, and pepper.

Fill mushroom caps with the spinach and goat cheese mixture.

Bake in the oven for 15-20 minutes or until mushrooms are tender and cheese is melted.

19. Citrus and Herb Baked Tilapia:

Ingredients:

4 tilapia fillets

Juice of 1 orange

Juice of 1 lime

2 tablespoons chopped fresh cilantro

2 tablespoons chopped fresh parsley

1 tablespoon olive oil

2 cloves garlic, minced

Salt and pepper to taste

Preparation:

Preheat the oven to 375°F (190°C).

In a bowl, mix orange juice, lime juice, chopped cilantro, chopped parsley, minced garlic, olive oil, salt, and pepper.

Marinate tilapia fillets in the mixture for 15-30 minutes.

Place tilapia fillets on a baking sheet and bake for 10-12 minutes or until fish is flaky and cooked through.

20. Lentil and Quinoa Stuffed Bell Peppers:

Ingredients:

4 large bell peppers, seeded and cut in half.

1 cup cooked lentils

1 cup cooked quinoa

1 cup diced tomatoes

1/2 cup chopped fresh parsley

1 tablespoon olive oil

1 teaspoon ground cumin

1 teaspoon smoked paprika

Salt and pepper to taste

Preparation:

Preheat the oven to 375°F (190°C).

In a large bowl, mix cooked lentils, cooked quinoa, diced tomatoes, chopped fresh parsley, olive oil, ground cumin, smoked paprika, salt, and pepper.

Fill each bell pepper half with the lentil and quinoa mixture.

Place stuffed bell peppers on a baking sheet and bake for 20-25 minutes until the peppers are tender.

21. Chicken and Vegetable Curry:

Ingredients:

1 pound of cut-up, skinless, boneless chicken breasts

1 cup of chopped, multicolored bell peppers

1 cup chopped zucchini

1 cup chopped carrots

1 can (14 oz) coconut milk

2 tablespoons curry powder

2 cloves garlic, minced

1 tablespoon grated ginger

2 tablespoons olive oil

Fresh cilantro for garnish

Salt and pepper to taste

Preparation:

Gently warm olive oil in a spacious skillet over medium-high heat.

Add chicken pieces, garlic, and grated ginger. Cook until chicken is browned.

Stir in curry powder, chopped bell peppers, zucchini, and carrots. Let the vegetables cook until they reach a delightful tender-crisp texture.

Pour in coconut milk and let the mixture simmer for 10-15 minutes until the sauce thickens.

Make sure to adjust the seasoning with salt and pepper according to your taste.

Garnish with fresh cilantro before serving.

22. Roasted Asparagus with Lemon and Parmesan:

Ingredients:

1 bunch asparagus, trimmed

2 tablespoons olive oil

Zest of 1 lemon

1/4 cup grated Parmesan cheese

Salt and pepper to taste

Preparation:

Preheat the oven to 400°F (200°C).

Place trimmed asparagus on a baking sheet. Drizzle some more olive oil over the dish and give it a good toss for an even coating.

Roast in the oven for 10-15 minutes or until asparagus is tender and slightly crispy.

Sprinkle with lemon zest, grated Parmesan, salt, and pepper before serving.

23. Shrimp and Avocado Salad:

Ingredients:

1 pound of peeled and deveined big shrimp

2 avocados, peeled and diced

1 cup cherry tomatoes, halved

1/4 cup chopped red onion

2 tablespoons chopped fresh cilantro

Juice of 1 lime
2 tablespoons olive oil

Salt and pepper to taste

Preparation:

In a large bowl, combine peeled and deveined shrimp, diced avocados, halved cherry tomatoes, chopped red onion, and chopped fresh cilantro.

In a separate bowl, whisk together fresh lime juice, olive oil, salt, and pepper to make the dressing.

Drizzle dressing over the shrimp and avocado mixture and toss to coat.

24. Cauliflower Crust Margherita Pizza:

Ingredients:
For the crust:

1 medium cauliflower head, grated

1 large egg

1 cup shredded mozzarella cheese

1 teaspoon dried oregano

Salt and pepper to taste

For the toppings:

1/2 cup marinara sauce

1 cup sliced cherry tomatoes

1 cup fresh basil leaves

1/2 cup shredded mozzarella cheese

Preparation:

Preheat the oven to 425°F (220°C).

Take the grated cauliflower and place it in a microwave-safe bowl, then microwave it for 5 minutes.

Let the cauliflower cool slightly, then squeeze out any excess water using a clean kitchen towel.

In a bowl, mix cauliflower, egg, shredded mozzarella, dried oregano, salt, and pepper to make the crust.

Spread the crust mixture onto a parchment-lined baking sheet and shape it into a round pizza crust.

Bake the crust in the oven for 15-20 minutes until it becomes firm and golden.

Remove the crust from the oven and top it with marinara sauce, sliced cherry tomatoes, fresh basil leaves, and shredded mozzarella cheese.

Pop the pizza back into the oven and bake it for an extra 10 minutes, until the cheese turns beautifully melted and bubbly.

25. Berry and Spinach Smoothie:

Ingredients:

1 cup fresh spinach leaves

1 cup containing a variety of berries, including strawberries, blueberries, and raspberries.

1 ripe banana

1 cup of almond milk or any milk you prefer.

1 tablespoon honey (optional)

Preparation:

In a blender, combine fresh spinach leaves, mixed berries, ripe banana, and almond milk.

Blend until smooth and creamy.

If desired, sweeten with honey.

Pour into a glass and enjoy a refreshing and nutritious smoothie.

Explore a collection of 25 Gout Diet recipes with a delightful range of flavors and ingredients, perfect for maintaining a gout-friendly lifestyle. Savor a healthy and enjoyable

culinary experience through this diverse assortment of dishes!

CONCLUSION

The Healthy Gout Diet Cookbook offers more than a simple collection of recipes; it presents a transformative journey towards embracing a life of wellness and culinary enchantment. Within its pages, a world of exquisite flavors dances harmoniously with gout-friendly ingredients, proving that health-conscious meals need not sacrifice taste or pleasure. This culinary adventure takes us from the quaint village of Goutville to our very own kitchens, celebrating the richness of nature's bounty and the artistry of gastronomy.

At the heart of each recipe lies the essence of passion and dedication, stemming from the personal journey of the beloved chef, Arthur. His determination to overcome the challenges of gout has led to the creation of these delectable dishes, which bring joy and nourishment to all who indulge in them.

Beyond being a mere guide to managing gout, this cookbook serves as an invitation to redefine our relationship with food. It encourages a harmonious balance between indulgence and well-being, showcasing that wholesome eating can be a source of delight rather than deprivation. With each meticulously crafted recipe, readers discover that nourishing their bodies can be a deeply gratifying and soul-enriching experience.

Yet, the journey doesn't end with the final page; it is a lifelong commitment to embracing the goodness that nature has to offer. As we venture forth into our culinary endeavors, this cookbook becomes a trusted companion, guiding us towards vibrant health and culinary mastery.

The hope is that this book inspires readers to unleash their creativity in the kitchen, infusing each meal with love and mindfulness, and sharing the joy of gout-friendly feasts with their loved ones. As the flavors are savored, the aromas relished, and the nourishment appreciated, it's essential to remember that the journey to better health and gastronomic delight begins within these very pages.

Let the cookbook be your guide to vibrant health and culinary mastery. May it inspire you to be creative in the kitchen, infuse love and mindfulness into each meal, and share gout-friendly feasts with loved ones. As you enjoy the flavors and aromas, remember that this is the beginning of a journey to better health and culinary joy. Thank you for joining us on this savory expedition. Embrace the art of gout-friendly cooking and may your culinary voyage be delightful, nourishing, and uplifting. Cheers to your health, joy, and culinary legacy. Bon appétit!